Greta Logan

Natural
Hair Care
Recipes

Amazing recipes to make your own natural homemade lotions for beauty and care of your hair

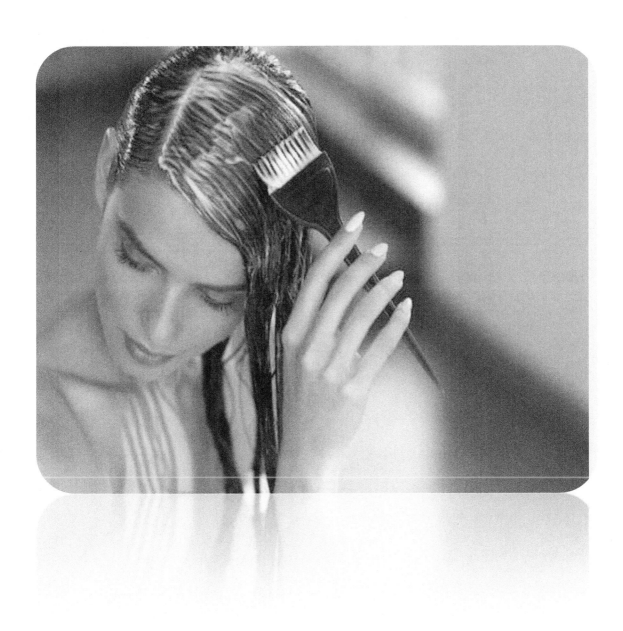

Table of Contents

Everything You Need to Know About Your Hair

LIFE EXPECTANCY OF HAIR

The life expectancy of hair is hereditary and usually ranges from two to seven years. In addition, 90% of the hair on the head regularly develops (known as the anagen phase) and 10% rest (known as the telogen phase). The length of the hair lasts about seven years, while medium-length hair lasts only about three years. In this way, only some individuals with long anagen times can hope to grow their hair up to the trunk. With age, the stage of development is shortened. For example, someone with a five-year development phase can develop hair to a length of about 2 feet before they enter the resting phase. If their development period falls to three years, while they are aging, their hair at this point becomes significantly half the length before it falls or is brushed. It is not unexpected to lose about 100 hairs a day from the scalp.

COMPOSITION OF HAIR

There are more than 12 different structures that make up each hair fiber. These structures make the hair a built-in structure that can demonstrate both independently and cooperatively. However, hair can be more effective, having only two structures: the cuticle (outside) and the cortex (inside). The hair fiber is made similar to a tree, with a layered exterior and a muscular interior. The skin of the nails is the guarantee of hair from the climate. It is made of solid protein and looks like a tile on the roof. The cortex is mainly responsible for the strength and body of the hair.

On the head of a normal individual, there are about 100,000 hairs. Since hair develops at a normal rate of 1 cm/month, in the hope that it was not conceivable to keep all the hair on his head from beginning to end, it will grow the sum of 100 feet for each day.

FOR WHAT REASON DOES AGE AFFECT THE SURFACE OF THE HAIR?

Dr. Elma Titus, trichologist at the trichology center in Cape Town, clarifies that such variables as chemotherapy, trauma, major activities, start or stop prescription, and long-range substance/mechanical damage will cause premature hair bad luck. The hairs complete the anagen-catagen-telogen cycle too quickly, and the new hairs have a better and more curious surface.

In addition, Titus warns: "the surface of the hair changes in the hope of not getting the basic nutrition from the inside."

The most effective way to treat hair surface changes

Titus suggests including amino acids that are found in proteins in your diet routine. The absence of protein creates less energy for the formation of cells—it involves cells engaged in hair development. She says, "breakfast is the main dinner for your hair because the energy levels [at your follicles are lowest] in the early part of the day."

WHAT CAUSES THINNING AT THE TOP?

Upper dilution is more normal in men than in women. Testosterone in men is used in dihydrotestosterone (DHT), which affects the follicle and the root. Titus clarifies the male example by decreasing (MPT): "with each new cycle, the affected hair does not develop longer and improves when measured. In the long run, fine hair remains. "In women, the ovaries and adrenal glands produce androgens. The spread of androgens can provoke a decrease in hereditary hair in women.

Treatment of hair thinning treatment

Local balm

Minoxidil

Finasteride.

Meso Treatment.

Stem cell treatment.

Treatment with light, laser, infrared.

Platelet-rich plasma (PRP) and

Scalp strips.

Titus prescribes blood tests to check for pallor since iron affects the work of the follicle. Iron is one of the main minerals for hair, along with zinc, copper, magnesium, calcium and nutrients D, B12 and B6. It proposes to control the pressure, as well as improve the nutrients containing minerals and key nutrients.

Natural Hair Care Recipes

Sound sparkling braids are each woman's dream. With new, costly hair items being dispatched ordinary, one thinks it's hard to pick the correct hair care item. With unreasonable utilization of synthetically planned items like shampoos, conditioners, colors, and so forth, the natural oils present in our hair and scalp are stripped off without any problem. For a lush head of solid hair while setting aside cash, give a portion of the underneath referenced natural hair care recipes at attempt— you will not be frustrated.

Back rub a very much beaten egg into newly washed hair. Wash it with cold water following five minutes. Keep away from high temp water, or more than likely, you will have fried eggs in your hair.

Mayo is an incredible hair conditioner. Back rub it completely and flush it carefully in virus water. High temp water will set the mayonnaise in your hair, so maintain a strategic distance from it.

Give your hair the last flush with not all that solid smelling lager to get a flawless sparkle.

Daintily heat the rosemary oil, knead it on to the scalp and let it sit for a few minutes prior to washing it off with warm water.

If the bothersome scalp is your concern, apply some yogurt. Wrap your hair with a towel for 15 minutes and afterward wash. Yogurt will pursue away dandruff as well.

Blend three pieces of water to one piece of vinegar; douse or shower your hair in this answer to eliminate any shampoo development. Wash as common, and you will discover that hair is anything but difficult to oversee and style.

Basic oils like ylang will invigorate hair development and go about as hair rejuvenator whenever added to one or the other shampoo or conditioner.

Washing your hair with the juice of 2-3 lemons will take sparkle back to the dull hair.

Homemade conditioner recipe. Apply a glue made with pounded avocados and mayonnaise for 15 minutes for the most extreme impact. Cover your head for 15-20 minutes and wash it off with a delicate shampoo.

For a sustaining hair conditioner, attempt this - heat three tbsp of coconut oil and 1/2 cup jojoba oil on low warmth.

Make a smooth glue with four tbsp powdered white dirt and one cup of water. Join the oils and white mud glue appropriately. Apply it on hosed and clean hair, rubbing it onto the scalp. Cover for 15 minutes and shampoo from that point. Jojoba oil utilized in hair care relaxes the scalp skin and gives additional sparkle and bob.

To trim the oil of slick hair, add a couple ofjuice vinegar tbsp during the last wash.

Olive oil is a great conditioner for dry hair. Back rub your hair altogether, particularly the closures and middles. Fold a warm towel over your head for 30 minutes, as the oil will enter the hair shaft. At that point, wash it, utilizing a delicate dry hair shampoo.

In the wake of washing your hair, wash it with some milk and let it sit for 15 minutes or something like that. Flush off with warm water to get the sheer quality and natural sparkle.

For sleek hair, beat one egg white and apply it on dry hair. Leave it till it dries and gets dry. Wash it off with cold water and shampoo. This will help lessens the sleekness whenever done routinely.

If your hair is harmed, attempt this pack. Blend juice of two newly crushed lemons, two egg yolks, one egg white and a tbsp of nectar. Apply onto the hair and let it rest for quite a while. Shampoo and flush off with cold water.

Natural Hair Care Homemade Recipes

If you have evaluated the expense of excellent hair items, at that point, you know there are many dollars to be spared by Natural Hair Care Homemade Recipes. It is not only for the in-your-face do it without anyone else's help people. Many of the recipes are age-old and still utilized today, even in luxurious salons. We should take a gander at certain methods for blending, applying, and the recipes themselves.

Innovative Mixing: Start with straightforward recipes. Blend one fundamental fixing and afterward add a limited quantity of another. It is a lot simpler to figure out what does constantly work when your fixings list.

Make blends and attempt them until you discover one that functions admirably for your hair. In the event that it's a formula that gives you incredible outcomes, cause note of it and afterward to retry the formula with a similar primary fixing yet now change the subsequent fixing to refine and modify the equation. You may discover you need to invert the fixings measures utilized, exchanging the principle fixing with the optional fixing.

Stunts for Applying: Experiment with applying your natural hair care natively constructed formula to your wet and dry hair. Likewise, explore different avenues regarding leaving it in your hair short-term. If you can eat it, it is likely protected in your hair. Better recipes can be spritzed on as a supplement coat for sparkle and body.

Recipes to build body and sparkle:

One medium ready avocado - stripped and stoned

Two tablespoons delicate nectar

Combine the fixings in a little bowl.

Back rub into hair.

Leave in for 20-30 minutes.

Wash hair as you ordinarily do.

Four egg whites

One pack kelp doused for the time being

One lemon crushed for juice

Combine the fixings in a blender.

Back rub into hair.

Leave in for 20-30 minutes.

Wash hair as you typically do.

4 Tablespoons Organic Coconut Oil liquefied at room temperature

Four drops of fundamental oil of your decisions, for example, peppermint or lavender

Combine the fixings in a little bowl.

Back rub into hair.

Leave in for an overnight

Wash hair as you typically do.

Other recommended fixings: Herbs can be applied from a tea - Comfrey Root, Calendula, Nettles, and Horsetail are brilliant tonics on the hair and are promptly accessible in most natural food stores. There are endless potential outcomes in utilizing Natural Hair Care Homemade Recipes. You may wish to likewise try different things with recipes for featuring. Additionally, you can stop hair misfortune at home utilizing these elements for silver hair natural cures. In addition to utilizing these recipes, make sure to brush your hair twice day by day, both forward and in reverse. Have a decent hair day and play around with your blends.

Make Your Own Incredible Shampoo

The hair care business, especially shampoos, has developed aesthetically. There are many brands, different shampoos and each specific for a single type of hair. Of all the expositions and targeted advertising around extraordinary shampoos, it is justifiable that shampoo has picked up some misconceptions about what it is and how to use it. To simplify, we will make the basics of shampoo for you, so the next time you use shampoo or buy another jar, you will settle for an informed choice and get the best shampoo for your hair.

These days, shampoo recipes will guarantee you everything from better shading to smoother surfaces or make your hair straighter and be faster. However, what a decent shampoo should do first is perfect for scalp and hair bolts. Basic and clear, and everything else that accompanies them is special rewards.

WHAT SHOULD SHAMPOO DO

Any recipe for shampoo before monetary delivery is widely concentrated by magnificence labs. Experts will try to make a shampoo recipe that will then be able to be a magnet for oils and junk while figuring out how to keep water and fend off those unwanted oils and wrecks and jetsam. In this way, your hair will be clean and maintain its regular appearance.

In addition to the ability to clean, there are different opinions that shampoo experts do not forget while making their ideal shampoo recipes. Above all, shampoo should not aggravate the eyes, scalp or skin, should not damage the hair in any position, and should be convincing in different types of water, from tap to water.

In your shampoo bottle, you will discover names such as Lauroamphoacetate chloride, obtained from coconut oil, and make your shampoo tear-free. It helps balance citric acid, which is an extreme aggravation removed from citrus soil products used to store oil in your shampoo and as a cancer prevention agent.

HOW SHAMPOO WORKS

Let's start by clarifying the problem. Like any other, your head produces oils designed to protect the hair and are very useful for the scalp. In any case, these oils will continue to move through the hair, and soon they will turn out to be smooth, sticky and undesirable. However, it will collect all kinds of cleaning products, garbage and dead skin. Another problem with these common oils is that they repel water. In case you have ever made a puncture while using only water to clean your hair, you will realize that it does not work so well.

At the time of applying shampoo, it will act much like a vacuum cleaner, which drives the entire soil and washes it with water. So, it is important that you require a long back massage with shampoo; in this way, it will allow you to compose all the ground and give time for the shampoo to use some other magnificence care elements in mind for its recipe. In addition, hair washing is a significant stage in the use of shampoo, as it eliminates the whole country, and the subsequent shampoo gives up.

You should use just enough shampoo to measure your hair; in this way, washing will be easier since there will not be much shampoo. After rinsing the hair with clean water, it is perfect and ready to dry. Along these lines, the basics of shampoos are covered, and next time you take a look at the bottle of shampoo, you will have a great deal of what goes for each day of care for your hair.

HOW TO USE DRY SHAMPOO AND SAVE TIME FROM WASHING YOUR HAIR

Knowing how to use dry shampoo can save a lot of time and effort. Dry shampoos are especially useful in the crazy morning hours of the working day when you need to rush to the workplace or carry out morning activities, and certainly do not have an ideal opportunity to wash the mop. Your shampoo powder can ingest an abundance of oil and soil that makes your locks dull and limp. It also removes the smell of unwashed hair and gives the volume of braids and jumps.

However, there is a science of using dry shampoo for hair. Excess from it will make your hair dull. Too little will make your locks unkempt. Also, hoping to use some unacceptable kind of shampoo powder, it will seem too obvious that you have not washed your hair. So, how would you use shampoo powder? Browse on and find out.

1. Consider the shade of your braids when choosing a shampoo powder. If you have light hair, you can use an unpainted dry shampoo. The powder is mixed directly into the hair. In the event that you have darker locks, you may need to use a colored shampoo, the shade of which coordinates the hue of the hair. In doing so, you will not

have to emphasize the pieces of shampoo that appear in your braids if you completely neglected them.

2. If it is not possible to determine the color of dry shampoo, which intensively coordinates the hair's tone, feel free to use non-colored powder shampoo. In any case, you should make some extra effort in making sure you have enough dust from the mop before leaving the bathroom.

3. Before applying dry shampoo to the scalp and hair, wash your hands thoroughly. With clean hands, you will not add earth and oil, which are already in your braids.

4. On the off chance that your shampoo powder arrives in an air container, spray the shampoo directly onto your foundation. In the event that you use a common space, load it in the palm of your hand. One tablespoon of shampoo is usually enough to clean the scalp and roots.

5. Rub the scalp with your fingertips. This will ensure that the dry shampoo will ingest the abundance of sebum and earth in your pigtails. Continue to rub the scalp until the dry shampoo completely breaks down.

6. Brush your hair. Brushing removes any shampoo powder left in the hair. Similarly, keep the hair shiny and smooth the entire knot from the locks.

7. Apply the hair conditioner to the base. The conditioner will give the hair shine and volume. It will also give your foundation and scalp the supplements they need to maintain your hair's soundness. Do not forget to apply the conditioner only to the base foundation. An abundance of conditioner will make your hair soft and heavy.

8. Adjust your hair as you need. If your hair looks dull, put a little hair serum on the hair's surface and only on the caps.

Dry shampoo is a very useful item you should have if you are regularly too busy to even consider washing your hair. Realizing how to use dry shampoo and having the right element for your hair, you can appreciate clean hair for a long time.

MAKE YOUR OWN SHAMPOO

Make your own shampoo? You may have never even thought about this, however truly, it is conceivable to make your own shampoo, and it's simple as well! You simply need a couple of straightforward, all-normal fixings to make this bubbly hair chemical. It works extraordinary, and you will set aside cash over business forms too. You can alter it to smell simply the way that you like it too.

Make your own shampoo by utilizing a formula that uses a normal Castile cleanser. Castile cleanser is 100% gotten from plant sources. Initially, Castile cleanser was made continuously with olive oil; in any case, there are different sorts accessible now that are obtained from hemp and other regular oils. You can either utilize a fluid Castile or a ground bar of a similar item for your shampoo formula. You could make your own Castile cleanser without any preparation in the event that you are truly committed; nonetheless, making a fluid cleanser without any preparation is a troublesome, tedious cycle for even experienced cleanser creators.

When you make your own shampoo, you are shielding yourself from synthetics regularly added to business shampoos. One extremely dubious fixing in many, if not most, business adaptations are sodium lauryl sulfate (SLS). This synthetic was initially planned as a motor degreaser. SLS is remembered for an assortment of skin and body care items on account of its amazing frothing activity and how it is exceptionally cheap. While SLS isn't a cancer-causing agent all alone, it is accepted to can join with different fixings in skincare items and hazardous structure nitrites, which have been connected to malignancy.

Make your own shampoo unique by altering the consistency, aroma, and helpful properties of your item. If you like a thicker shampoo, add less water when making it; or add more water if you like a slender item. You can add basic oils for both an incredible, new fragrance and helpful characteristics. For instance, rosemary fundamental oil can be added to help control slick hair or basic lavender oil for those with a delicate scalp.

The most troublesome advance when you make your own shampoo is grinding up the Castile cleanser. On the off chance that you can deal with that and do a touch of liquefying over boiling water, at that point, you have all the aptitudes you require to make your own, stand-out shampoo made only the manner in which you like it. As buyers, we have been conned by huge hair care organizations that this is a troublesome errand and past our aptitudes when nothing could be further from reality.

Just endeavor to register the sum you spend on shampoo in a year's time, and you will quickly come to recognize how much shampoo we truly use! Just imagine making your own shampoos in the fragrance and consistency that YOU need. I will pass on a few designs for a shampoo that you will truly venerate, so set up; the main will be anything but not difficult to make.

The essential shampoo is dry shampoo, and the result will stun you. The trimmings that you will require include:

1/2 cup cornstarch

Smell oil (optional)

Sprinkle cornstarch into your hair and back rub into hair and scalp. License it to ingest for a few minutes; by then, brush through hair. Repeat if fundamental. This is incredible to tidy up your hair when totally fundamental between shampoos. It is then uncommon to go on outside excursions when freshwater is difficult to reach for using liquid shampoo. Moreover, you can add a few drops of smell oil to the cornstarch for a lovely scented dry shampoo.

Next, we will explore a more trademark shampoo known as Egg Shampoo, and you will require:

One egg

1 tsp. olive oil

1 tsp. lemon juice

1 T. Castile chemical or delicate unscented shampoo

1/2 C. water

Join all trimmings in a blender and whip until smooth. Use shampoo rapidly, and find a hair wash. Save any abundance of shampoo in the cooler and use it the next day.

Another trademark grouping fuses Lemon-Egg Shampoo, which is astonishing for ricochet and shimmer and the once-over of things required are:

1 egg

1 tsp. lemon juice

3 tbs. unscented shampoo

Fragrance oil of your choice

Unite all trimmings in a bowl. Shampoo into your hair and wash well.

The egg will probably go as a conditioner, and the lemon juice will convey an attempt to satisfy hair!

One of my undisputed top decisions consolidate a local shampoo which is essentially for smooth hair, and it joins:

2 tbs. dry peppermint

2 tbs. dry spearmint

1 tbs. dry sage

1 cup of water

2/3 cup kid shampoo

Unite flavors and water in a pot and warmth to the point of bubbling. Kill from warmth and license to drench for 20 minutes. Strain out the flavors and mix the baby shampoo with the local water. Fill a plastic spray container or holder.

After a good washing, forming is the accompanying stage, and here are two or three designs for customary conditioners that are remarkable for the strength of your hair; let us start with:

Nectar Herbal Hair Conditioner

1/4 cup nectar

1/4 cup glycerin

1/4 cup sage and 1/2 cup dried chamomile blooms

Or then again

1/2 cup pester leaves and 1/4 cup rosemary leaves

1/2 cup witch hazel

1 tablespoon liquid lecithin

Detect everything on the side in a screw-top compartment. Shake well and let sit for an hour. Strain to dispense with flavors, discard the flavors, and void the liquid back into the compartment. Makes around 1/2 cup.

If you are bothered with smooth hair and need assistance speedy, by then you should have a go at using Honey-Milk Conditioner for Oily Hair and the trimmings include:

1/3 cup high temp water

¼ cup glycerin

2 tablespoons liquid lecithin

1/4 cup Sage

1/4 cup nectar

2 tablespoons dry buttermilk powder

Unite the high temp water and sage, and set for 10 minutes. Strain the liquid, and discard the sage. Add the overabundance trimmings to the focused on liquid, and mix well. Apply to recently shampooed hair, let set on hair for around 2 minutes, and flush off with warm water. Makes around 1/2 cup.

I do have an admonition on the off chance that you are shading your hair: you risk your shading blurring or, in any event, being eliminated when you utilize these natively constructed items. Before you use any of these on shaded hair, you will need to test them on some hair that is moderately covered up.

Apple Cider Vinegar

We overall are searching for a thing that does some extraordinary things. Whether or not it be for skincare, prosperity, or hair care, there is a consistent requirement for a thing that can finally discard our defects and let our eminence shimmer. Luckily, a thing, for instance, this is not a legend. Squeezed apple vinegar, an all basic thing, helps with liberating the skin of skin aggravation, helps weight decrease, and assuages dry and feeble hair.

Skincare

This vinegar is an unprecedented skincare thing. It can discard skin aggravation, clear up old blemishes, and help to shed dead skin. Other skin irritation medications use savage manufactured mixes and consistently dry out the skin. As squeezed apple vinegar is acidic, it helps with isolating the oils, causing skin irritation. To use, you can either make a squeezed apple vinegar wash or simply apply it from the container onto a cotton ball.

As a flush, 1 or 2 tablespoons of squeezed apple vinegar should be mixed in with 1 to 1/2 cups of water. In the wake of using your standard face chemical, flush your face with the mix. The vinegar smell may not be pleasurable from the outset yet will subside within 15 minutes. Notwithstanding how you don't have to debilitate the vinegar, it is fundamental to use unrefined, unadulterated squeezed apple vinegar. In case it is arranged in one way or another, it won't be adequate even undiluted for your regular use.

Weight decrease

It is a remarkable alternative to the various unsafe and unapproved weight decrease pills accessible. It is an all trademark thing that has essentially zero pernicious effects. At whatever point used suitably, it is harmless. For deferred use, it should be debilitated considering its acidic properties. Else, it is harmless.

There have not been various assessments done to reason that squeezed apple vinegar alone is a helpful manual for weight decrease. The vast majority of experts who have done examinations acknowledge that the thing is valuable, considering that it helps the stomach related cycle, which helps the subject feel full speedier. Others acknowledge that since it is ingested in a water mix preceding eating, the liquid itself is simply finishing off the stomach snappier. Regardless, various people have viably shed pounds with its use. To use it as a weight decrease, debilitate 1 to 2 tablespoons in a water container. Drink the mix inside 30 minutes before your supper.

Hair Care

It is also perhaps best used for hair care. Various shampoos have silicone or are stacked with sulfate. Sulfates dry out the hair and can wrap up creation the hair dry. This is the principal purpose of using a conditioner after shampoo. Silicone adds greater advancement to hair, which essentially invalidates the purpose of shampooing, regardless. For those looking for more useful ways to deal with care for their hair, consider changing to a squeezed apple vinegar wash for shampoo. If you shampoo every day, use the squeezed apple vinegar wash and simply your customary shampoo once consistently. This may be changed depending upon how much soil and advancement you total on your scalp.

This thing works for hair correspondingly; it works for various vocations. From its basic, acidic properties, it isolates the oil and soil on the scalp and hair. Despite being a trademark substance, it loosens up hair moreover. For those with dry and feeble hair wanting to smooth hair, use a squeezed apple vinegar flush around 2 to multiple times every week. This is perhaps the one Steps of squeezed apple vinegar where it should not be debilitated, so a great deal if it's no different to you the smell. If you do, debilitate comparably like you were to wash your face or drink for weight decrease.

ROSEMARY WASHING HAIR

Pay attention to the distant option of having light blond hair because rosemary can darken. This washing will make your hair blink on the chance that you darken on light brown hair. Boil two tablespoons of dry rosemary in a cup of water and add two tablespoons of almond oil and a quarter teaspoon of lemon oil. Wash your hair and rinse well.

PREPARATION OF SODA SHAMPOO

The soda preparation has gained notoriety for removing stains and dirt and is the same as for hair. Things come out; nothing develops on the hair, including gel, foam, conditioner, and hairspray. Use it sparingly, however, on more than one occasion per month, probably. This product can actually dry the hair shaft; it can also break the skin of the nails when used regularly.

To use a warming drink for hair, combine one and a half teaspoons with half a cup of warm water. Place in a small plastic container and shake for a long time before use. Back rub a limited amount into the scalp and along the hair shaft for caps. Wash well.

RASSOUL CLAY HAIR CLEANSER

On the off chance that you need something a little extravagant for your hair, try this one. Rassoul mud comes from the irregular locals of Morocco and continues forever. The earth is smooth to the touch and is charged with minerals. This chemical eliminates the breakdown of hair and scalp-dandruff and all-while saturating the hair shaft.

You can make this chemical for hair by combining three tablespoons of mud with enough water to make glue. Add a teaspoon of almond oil to the mixture and mix well. Again, rub this glue into the hair, and the scalp is not moisturized. Leave for three to five minutes before taking a step in the shower and wash. This chemical does some amazing things for damaged and dry hair.

CORN FLOUR CLEANER CHINA MANUFACTURER

You can use this powder if you do not have the opportunity to wash your hair. Removes earth and oils from everything except greasy hair.

To prepare this chemical, consolidate a tablespoon of salt with half a cup of cornflour and put it in a shaker container. To use it, rub a little light on your hair and brush through and out to get rid of dirt and oil. This is an approach to making your hair noticeably immaculate without water.

Coconut Oil

Coconut oil is enormous in Asia and the Caribbean and is quickly jumping on in various countries. Coconut oil is one of the most renowned oils to use for hair. The oil begins as a solid and must be warmed, either from the glow of your hands and fingers or in a compartment. An excellent natural conditioner, coconut oil can be used alone, blended in with various oils, or, as often as possible, a base for a hair recipe. For the best results, use virgin coconut oil since it isn't as ready and has more proteins.

The adaptable oil placates hair beginning at the shaft, invigorates, progresses hair improvement, and keeps the scalp unblemished and strong. It similarly smells magnificent!

COCONUT OIL SHAMPOO

Trimmings:

2 teaspoons virgin coconut oil

1 Tablespoon Castile chemical

1/2 cup refined water

Headings:

Mix trimmings in a container. Totals can be accustomed to make more shampoo. The recipe above is the norm. Shampoo with a mix as you routinely would.

COCONUT OIL CONDITIONER

Trimmings:

2 Tablespoons virgin coconut oil

1 Tablespoon almond oil

Headings:

1) Warm the coconut oil in a skillet to break it up. Add the almond oil and blend. Dispose of heat.

2) Coat hair from root to tip in the mix. Get hair into a shower cap and crease a hot towel over your head. License to warm through for 15-20 minutes.

*Tip: A towel warmed in the dryer for 15-20 minutes will be sufficiently warmed.

3) Rinse hair totally. Wash and condition hair consistently following treatment.

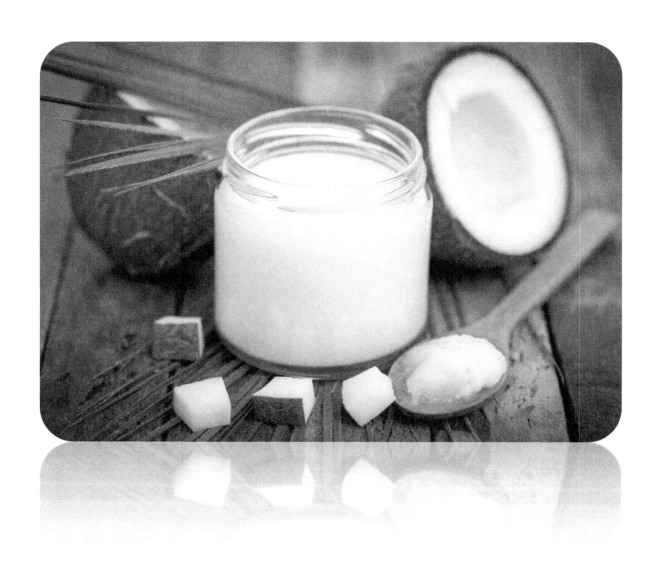

Essential Oils

Essential oils will be oils that have been removed from spices or blossoms and are exceptionally focused. These oils feed, ensure, and purify hair, animating new hair development. Normally, essential oil isn't applied without help from anyone else yet rather blended in with another oil. The most widely recognized essential oils utilized for hair development medicines are lavender, peppermint, rosemary, and tea tree.

ESSENTIAL OIL TREATMENT

Fixings:

1 cup almond oil

10 drops tea tree or peppermint oil

Headings:

Apply to hair starting at the scalp and working down to the tips of the hair. Cover hair with a shower cap and leave for washing with shampoo and molding for the time being.

Because of essential oils having anti-bacterial properties, profound scalp and hair medicines leave the hair more advantageous and fuller. The accompanying formula is for an incidental essential oil treatment:

PROFOUND SCALP CONDITIONER

Trimming:

1 Tablespoon olive oil

1 Tablespoon dim molasses

3 drops peppermint oil

1 egg

1/2 cup apple juice vinegar

Headings:

1) Combine all fixings aside from vinegar. In a crush bottle, consolidate the vinegar and 1 cup of warm water. Set in the shower to utilize later.

2) Wet hair with warm water.

3) Apply the conditioner to the hair from the root to the tip.

4) Wrap head in a hot towel. Let sit for 15 minutes.

*Note: be certain you utilize a towel that is old since molasses can recolor!

5) Rinse hair and shampoo completely.

6) Once the water runs neatly from the hair, utilize the vinegar flush as the last advance in the treatment.

Emu Oil

Standard in Australia, Emu oil isn't striking,except if you have sorted out some way to take a couple to get back some levelheadedness of a thing containing the oil. Stacked with Omega-3 unsaturated fats, the oil thickens, invigorates, and recovers hair advancement skin sicknesses. Your most intelligent decision is to find an Emu thing by methods for the web. Be vigilant; nonetheless, rough Emu oil can contain microorganisms that will make you incapacitated. Stick to refined Emu oil and related things.

If you can get your hands on Emu oil alone, simply use the oil as you would some other for oil treatment. Coat the hair from root to tip, cover with a shower cap, license to sit for at any rate an hour, anyway overnight would be ideal, flush inside and out, and wash hair.

Grandmother's Favorite Foaming Shampoo

This shampoo makes foam, yet it is delicate. The accompanying fixings make up the base.

In a plastic container, join:

1 ½ cup of water,

1 ½ cup of fluid Castile cleanser, and

1 ½ teaspoon of olive oil.

You can substitute Jojoba or grapeseed oil if you need an option that could be lighter than olive oil. Blend this up and store it in a shut plastic holder. I would recommend adding a couple of drops of essential oil for a refreshing scent. If you have an irritated or scaling scalp, add a couple of drops of tea tree oil. Lavender oil and lemon oil function admirably for slick hair; these are astringents that trim down on the oil your body produces.

You don't need to add essential oils that will really "accomplish something." If you appreciate apples or strawberries' fragrance, add a couple of drops of those essential oils to the shampoo. It will wait in your hair after it is washed. My number one scents are a combination of apricot and pineapple.

Natural Hair Conditioners

It has become a significant pattern in the present social orders to search for natural items instead of artificially man-made items. Excellence gracefully is the same as cleaning supplies, working supplies, or some other flexibility you may need, and natural hair conditioners are becoming famous in the present market. Gradually, natural hair conditioners are ascending their way to the highest point of the hair care stepping stool as they assist you with keeping up solid, lovely, and pubescent hair while utilizing every natural item, so you don't need to contemplate whether your hair will consume off or whatever else like that. Individuals today are becoming ill of the powerlessness to articulate the synthetic compounds found in the items they are utilizing in their hair. They are tired of thinking about how their hair will respond. With natural hair conditioners, your hair will remain protected and solid; all things considered, nobody has ever known about lemon juice, making their hair drop out, right?

The vast majority do not understand the unforgiving impacts of a portion of the items they are utilizing in their hair today, and that shouldn't be valid. Did you realize that our hair's natural oils contain nutrients and minerals that are more beneficial than most man-made minerals out there? That is why shampoo is so horrible for your hair; it strips away the entirety of nature's purities and leaves your hair void, which is why most shampoos recommend the utilization of conditioners. Conditioners were initially intended to fix the harm done by shampoos in any case, thus utilizing natural hair conditioners is a surprisingly better method of reestablishing those minerals to your hair and scalp than the man-made substance conditioners.

It is actual; specialists state there are no genuine motivations to utilize the shampoo in any case, so how would we keep our hair clean? It's basic; keeping your hair clean doesn't mean stripping it of each oil on your scalp. It basically implies freeing your hair of destructive microbes' so it's useful to do precisely that. There are items out there that comprise whole lines of purging conditioners; a portion of these are largely natural hair conditioners and are so useful for the hair you can get results in as long as seven days! These items are best since you can avoid the shampoo part altogether and still have clean solid hair without having hair deprived of its natural aiding specialists.

The best intention for apply natural hair conditioners into your daily practice and to guarantee you keep on having glad sound hair is to utilize natural hair shampoo too, this way you're getting the entire framework with no new advances or rules, and you realize your hair is as yet protected and all-natural eventually. So remember, when attempting to adopt an all-natural strategy to hair care, utilize your investigating abilities and hope to discover what's out there; who realizes you may really be shocked, some natural hair conditioners can, in reality, even be made in your kitchen!

TYPES OF HAIR CONDITIONER

The most well-known sort is the standard conditioner that arrives in a container and has a rich consistency. These conditioners normally join a shampoo of a similar brand and are intended for regular use. They are not thick and can be utilized consistently.

Hair conditioners are additionally accessible as medicines. These are hair-conditioner particularly planned for harmed hair and are extremely solid and supporting. They are intended to give profound sustenance to the hair to fix the harm. Generally, these conditioners are left in the hair short-term and cleaned out the following day.

Leave-in conditioner is additionally a typical kind of straightener. These are light conditioners that are intended to be left in the hair in the wake of washing and are not flushed out. This kind of hair conditioner is ideal for dry crimped hair as it makes hair smooth and smooth. You can undoubtedly discover a leave-in conditioner that is intended for your hair type. Leave-in conditioners are essential for individuals who warmth style their hair as it shields from harm.

You can pick any hair-straightener out of these, relying upon your sort and your necessities. On the off chance that you have dry and harmed hair,at that point, profound conditioners and medicines are essential for you. Something else, a standard conditioner or a leave-in conditioner, is adequate.

COMPOSITION AND ADVANTAGES OF HAIR CONDITIONERS

Natural oils are being used for quite a long time to condition dry and dull human hair. It frequently alludestoa thick fluid that is rubbed and applied to the hair. It is quite a stunning item thatchanges the appearance and surface of the hair. A quality hair conditioner may contain sunscreen, oils and, creams, along with some different fixings. It is commonly utilized in the wake of giving a wash to the hair with any shampoo.

Albeit natural oils have been utilized for quite a long time, hair molding, yet the advanced techniques for hair molding were presented in 1900 in Paris. The recently presented item could just give a delicate touch to men's hair, mustaches, and whiskers.

Lately, current innovation and examination had made it conceivable to present such hair conditioners that don't give any hefty or oily inclination to its client. These are made of smelling salts, alcohols, and silicone.

Different sorts of hair conditioners are accessible in the market nowadays, which are as per the following:

Conventional conditioners, which we can by and large apply straightforwardly to our body after utilizing a shampoo.

Leave-in conditioners are made of chains of unsaturated fats. These chains are less gooey and add a slenderer oily layer to the hair. Their thickness confers them slick qualities. It very well may be utilized simply like hair oil and keeps hair straight and smooth.

Hold conditioners, which work simply like gels and can keep your hair in a shape as you wish to give them.

Pack conditioners, which are incredibly gooey and exceptionally thought, these dilemmas the hair together and stick them as you wish to give an ideal shape to the hair and keep them unblemished for a more extended time. These are typically made of unsaturated fat chains, which add a thicker layer to the hair.

The main elements of hair conditioners may incorporate yet not restricted to oils, creams, and additives. They may likewise incorporate sunscreen, which ensures it against shading misfortune and corruption of protein atoms. The sunscreens utilized in hair conditioners are very extraordinary to those utilized in skin items. They are normally acidic; their causticity is all because of natural acids, such as citrus extract.

How significant hair molding is, simply envision the distinction between an infertile and a prolific land. A fruitless land is without any grass, plant, or tree, while a ripe land gives a lovely look with rich green plants, verdant scenes, and elegant plants and trees. The same is the distinction betweendry and dull hair and all around adapted hair. Our hair is regularly presented to the soil, contaminations, and hair shading synthetic substances. They make them inclined to harm and crimped look. A conditioner steps in to reestablish them back their life and shine.

Hair conditioners and shampoo generally go together. Shampoo fills in as a purging specialist, while conditioners secure and grant magnificence to the hair by covering a slender layer over the outside of the hair. The principle drawback of utilizing a shampoo habitually is that while purifying the earth of hair, layers of fingernail skin cover and ensure hair shafts, making hair powerless against harm and getting more fragile daintier. As opposed to this, a conditioner adds a flimsy layer of dampness to these fingernail skin and ensures hair.

Hair adds an excessive amount to magnificence and character. Sound hairs need an excessive amount of care and consideration. Numerous brisk home cures are accessible in the market to secure and give a wonderful look to your hair. Hair molding is one of them. You may plan and utilize them at the solace of your home or get them from a superstore. However, the fact is how to apply them in thebest way to accomplish the best outcomes.

In the end, a few words about natural conditioners. They have a similar effect on your hair as fake conditioners would have;maybe they can deliver better outcomes over those accessible in business sectors. They incorporate natural fixings, such as olive oil, eggs, yogurt, banana, and numerous others with no results by any stretch of the imagination. They are effectively accessible on the lookout and more financially savvy. Today, different naturally made conditioners are likewise accessible in the market that can set aside time and cash, or more all, they are better for your hair's soundness.

HOW TO APPLY HAIR CONDITIONER?

If you need to encounter the most extreme advantages of utilizing a hair conditioner, you should buy an item appropriate for your kind of hair; moreover, you should likewise know about the correct cycle of utilizing it. There are fundamentally two sorts of conditioners. The primary kind is intended for people who need to give their mane moment sparkle and perfection; if you are utilizing this sort, you should stand by just a short time prior to washing off the applied conditioner. The other kind is intended for individuals searching for profound molding. The profound molding arrangement will offer the best outcomes on the off chance that you keep your secures splashed for 45 minutes to 60 minutes. Molding arrangements can likewise be ordered dependent on the kind of hair they are intended for, for example, hair conditioners for dry hair, conditioners for slim hair and so forth. The main thing that is basic in every one of these items is their cycle of use.

Pick the Right Product or Making the Right Conditioner

Pick the molding arrangement that is explicitly intended for your sort of hair. Individuals with slender or fine bolts ought to consistently choose light conditioners. People with artificially harmed locks, then again, ought to go through a profound molding treatment. On the off chance that you have shaded hair, we would encourage you to utilize an item planned, especially shading treated locks. In any case, for best outcomes, remember to apply the profound molding answer for your hair at any rate once consistently.

If your twists are short, you should apply hair conditioners just if it is hued, harmed or dry. People with long hair, notwithstanding, ought to never miss their week after hair molding meet. An individual with long bolts can keep away from the use of hair molding specialists just in the event that the person has sleek hair.

Besides picking the correct molding answer for your locks, you should likewise pick the correct shampoo to encounter the most extreme advantages of going through a molding treatment if your hair is tolerably dry; consistently pair conditioners for dry hair with shampoos implied for people with ordinary hair. In any case, if your twists are unreasonably dry, both your shampoo and conditioner should be items intended for dry hair. Individuals utilizing conditioners implied for shading treated locks, then again, ought to consistently utilize shading securing shampoos.

Application Procedure

Stage 1: Wash your locks utilizing the correct shampoo and flush it completely. Presently, set it up for the molding meeting by eliminating overabundance of water utilizing a towel.

Stage 2: Take a satisfactory measure of conditioner and apply it fastidiously on your hair. Ensure that each hair is covered appropriately with the molding specialist.

Stage 3: Now, brush your locks utilizing a wide-toothed brush to permit the conditioner to spread equally.

Stage 4: If you are utilizing an ordinary conditioner, hang tight for 5 minutes and wash your hair off completely using tepid water. For individuals going through a profound molding treatment, the holding up time should be at any rate 45 minutes.

Stage 5: The last advance will expect you to run cool water over the treated bolts consistently for 30 seconds. That is it; when completely dried, your hair will be smoother and shinier than at any other time.

PAPAYA CONDITIONER

Papayas are ample in supplements and minerals that are helpful for your hair. Blended with yogurt, they make an impeccable conditioner for your hair that smells adequately charming to eat (and it is).

To make and use this heavenly mix, combine one prepared papaya with the skin wiped out and a half cup of plain yogurt. Work the stuff into your hair, cover it with a shower cap, and let it set for 30 minutes. After it has stewed well, wash everything out, flushing totally. If you make extra, you can, for the most part, have some for breakfast!

NECTAR CONDITIONER

Nectar is hard to get away from your hair, yet it is incredibly stable. It immerses and urges hair to hold in the sogginess. You should clean it out with more sultry water than is commonly used on hair. With this treatment, your hair won't be wonderful until it squeaks when you run it between your thumb and fingers.

You can make this nectar conditioner by whisking one tablespoon of nectar with a half cup of plain yogurt. Apply to hair and scalp, leave it on for two or three minutes, and after that, wash totally with warm water.

SQUASHED BANANA CONDITIONER

Bananas are stacked with potassium, and like avocados, they help to fix hurt hair. This conditioner is difficult to clean out to some degree, yet the preferences are unquestionably legitimized even despite the trouble.

To make this conditioner, squash a banana in a bowl and add two drops of almond oil (or olive oil). Apply to the hair and hold set up with a shower cap for around 20 minutes. Wash well, yet don't shampoo.

MAYONNAISE CONDITIONER

Mayonnaise contains eggs, vinegar, and oil, which can restore a hurt fingernail skin and thwart future damage. It is overflowing with protein and adds fortitude to hair strands.

To use mayonnaise as a hair conditioner, just apply an unobtrusive bundle of the stuff to your dry hair. Put on a shower cap and let it set for 20 minutes. Wash first, by then shampoo.

Saturating dry hair. To tame frizz and saturate dry hair, join an egg, a tablespoon of olive oil and a cup of yogurt. Blend sufficiently and knead this combination into your hair and scalp. Leave on for in any event an hour and afterward, shampoo it off your mind. You will see gentler, shinier hair after the main application. Rehash on more than one occasion for each month.

SUBDUING A SLEEK SCALP

In case you are burnt out on the level, slick hair, take a stab at blending some yogurt, an egg white and several drops of lime squeeze. Apply generously to your braids, covering your hair and scalp. The lime squeeze and egg whites will help with balancing out your hair without adding to more slickness.

PROBIOTIC RICHNESS

It is safe to say that you are beginning to see that yogurt's advantages go a long way past stomach-related well-being and sustenance? Have a go at utilizing whipped yogurt instead of your shampoo and conditioner a few times each week to both condition and wash your hair simultaneously.

PROTEIN AND CITRUS

To liven up dull hair and add sparkle, join an entire egg with two tablespoons of lemon juice. Leave the combination on your hair for 20 minutes. This molding treatment joins protein and citrus to add sparkle and life to dull braids.

HOT OIL GOODNESS

A week-by-week hot oil scalp treatment can help you keep up a serious shine sheen on your locks. Warm-up a couple of tablespoons of olive oil until it isn't exactly hot to the touch, and afterward, knead it uniformly and altogether over your hair and scalp. Enclose your head with plastic and cover with a hot towel. Leave the hot oil treatment on your hair for about 60 minutes; at that point, wash.

WONDERFUL HENNA

You've presumably known about henna for making Indian mehndi brief tattoos or as an all-natural hair color; notwithstanding, henna is likewise an amazing hair conditioner. To get its hair care benefits, blend some henna powder in with one egg and a tablespoon of lime juice. Add a touch of yogurt varying to streamline the combination so it very well may be spread over your hair. Apply the combination equally over hair and scalp and leave it on until it begins to dry and solidify a piece. Shampoo hair clean. Utilize this treatment once every month for ideal outcomes.

PROFOUND SCALP CONDITIONER

Ingredients:

1 Tablespoon olive oil

1 Tablespoon dim molasses

3 drops peppermint oil

1 egg

1/2 cup apple juice vinegar

Steps:

1) Combine all fixings aside from vinegar. In a crush bottle, consolidate the vinegar and 1 cup of warm water. Set in the shower to utilize later.

2) Wet hair with warm water.

3) Apply the conditioner to the hair from the root to the tip.

4) Wrap head in a hot towel. Let sit for 15 minutes.

*Note: be certain you utilize a towel that is old since molasses can recolor!

5) Rinse hair and shampoo completely.

6) Once the water runs neatly from the hair, utilize the vinegar wash as the last advance in the treatment.

ALOE LEAVE-IN CONDITIONER

Ingredients:

1/2 cup water

1/2 cup Aloe Vera gel

10 drops tea tree oil

Directions:

1) Mix ingredients in a spray bottle.

2) Spray in hair and comb to distribute. Great for detangling curls!

MAYO MASSAGE AND CONDITIONING TREATMENT

Ingredients:

Mayo (enough to cover all your hair and scalp)

*Note: Use mayonnaise with the full-fat substance. Try not to utilize low-calorie or low-fat renditions. You need all the fat to saturate your hair. It's not as though you will eat it!

Steps:

1) Wet hair, or you can wash hair. First, it is up to you. Press out any overabundance of water, so the hair is simply moist, however altogether wet. As such, no dry spots.

2) Spread the mayo through your hair from root to tip, working your fingers between the locks to cover each strand.

3) Wrap head in saran wrap.

4) Let the mayo absorb for around 30 minutes.

5) Rinsing alone will not get the mayo out, so wash your hair with a mellow shampoo. It may take two or three washings on the off chance that you have thick hair.

ROSEMARY HAIR CONDITIONER

Rosemary is supposed to be the best hotspot for hair development. Additionally, this is a viable solution for a bothersome scalp and dandruff and making your hair a lot milder, reasonable, and smelling pleasant.

Ingredients:

Rosemary essential oil

Sweet almond or olive oil (marginally warmed)

Technique:

Blend 2-5 drops of rosemary essential oil with one teaspoon of sweet almond or olive oil, mix them well. Presently apply the blended oil to your hosed hair and back rub the scalp tenderly. Envelop your head with a hot towel and hang tight for around 45 minutes, so it profoundly conditions your hair. Flush off with cold water.

Note: Keep away from getting at you.

Warning: If you are pregnant, at that point, maintain a strategic distance from this hair conditioner as this may cause hypertension or epilepsy assault.

PROFOUND CONDITIONER

Avocados contain are a rich wellspring of nutrients B6 and E

Ingredients:

1 little container of genuine mayonnaise

1/2 avocado

Technique:

Take a medium-sized bowl, put all the fixings in it and crunch along with your hands until it transforms into a minty green tone. Apply this conditioner easily into your hair right to the tips. What's more, after all, wrap a towel on your head or cover it with a shower cap.

Sit tight for 20 minutes. For better and more profound molding, wrap your head with a hot, sodden towel - over the plastic wrap. What's more, on the off chance that you are sufficiently fortunate to have long hair and need to profound condition at the finishes, at that point, trim all the fixings into half and apply to the closures and wrap them appropriately.

PROFOUND CONDITIONER

Ingredients:

1/2 cup of genuine mayonnaise

Strategy: Apply the genuine mayonnaise over your moist hair and sift through it through the hair. Presently, envelop your head with a towel, hang tight for 20 minutes, and afterward shampoo.

Alert: Use the genuine mayonnaise and NOT serving of mixed greens dressing. This Salad Dressing will make your hair dry.

Storage: There is a greater part of the recipes that should be refrigerated, yet that doesn't imply that there are additives in them. Their time of usability is around a multi-week.

HOW TO MAKE HAIR CONDITIONER WITH AN AVOCADO

In case you're considering how you can utilize an avocado to condition your hair, the accompanying data will assist you with doing it. A decent aspect regarding utilizing avocados as a hair conditioner is that if you open an avocado and notice it's dull or has an adjustment in flavor or has too many dark spots and you're awkward eating it, you can trim them out and use it as a conditioner, so it's not squandered. Utilize a natural avocado if you need a natural hair conditioner.

If you've never utilized an avocado as a hair conditioner treatment, I propose that you give around a shot a couple of strands of hair first - not long before you wash or shampoo your hair. That way, you'll know whether it'll clean out effectively. It should clean out effectively; however,it's more permeable on the off chance that you have blanched hair, and it very well might be somewhat harder to cleanout. Yet, as a rule, there is no issue cleaning it out. In any case, it's in every case great to test if you have any reservations.

OK - you have your avocados. I'm accepting you realize how to open them or eat them routinely or day by day as I do. I have eaten an avocado consistently for over nine years. Furthermore, I have extraordinary clear skin and sparkly hair.

I like to chop it down the center longwise and pull the two parts separately and scoop out the avocado pit. Wash your hands completely first.

Crush the avocado up completely in a little glass bowl utilizing a fork. You need it to be finished pounded, without any pieces appearing. Presently gather up your crushed avocado combination and work it into your hair utilizing simply warm water, never hot. Likewise, apply it to your scalp. If you have time and feel so slanted, apply it to your face too. It will dry quickly and feel like a veil. Simply think - no additives, added substances or other cruel synthetics! Just loads of phytonutrients.

Avocados are one of the world's absolute best nourishments. They contain a high measure of oil. They have an adjusted pH, so they are neither corrosive nor antacid. They are plentiful in minerals that manage body capacities. Eating avocados are best for your hair, skin, and assimilation. Avocados are an acceptable wellspring of fat AND protein. Indeed, many individuals do not understand there is protein in each food grown from the ground. They additionally have great measures of iron and copper.

Recollect that hair is dead and the best advantages will come from eating avocados. In case you are one of only a handful few individuals who do not care for avocados, you can have a go at eating them with a little sun-dried ocean salt and check whether that has any kind of effect. Or then again, eat guacamole.

Note—It takes around ten avocados to make one teaspoon of avocado oil, which can really hurt the liver; however, if you eat ten avocados, they will not hurt you. Avocado oil items are costly and ordinarily contain additives and different synthetic substances. You need not bother with them. You can do an avocado hair molding treatment once every month or at whatever point you locate an avocado you cannot utilize. Make a point to eat an avocado consistently for the most radiant skin and hair. It works from within shockingly better where it can chip away at hair follicles, skin, and numerous other body measures. You will discover your hair and skin shining and be always snared on avocados.

WHY ARE PEOPLE USING MAYONNAISE IN THEIR HOMEMADE HAIR CONDITIONERS?

There are many strategies in making your own special natively constructed hair conditioner and yes, utilizing mayonnaise is one of them!

Indeed, where do we start? I did not understand that individuals utilized mayonnaise and spread avocado on their hair until just as of late. The custom-made hair conditioner prevailing fashion is certainly a hit for many individuals in the hair business, yet in addition for individuals who need to take care of their hair at home.

From the exploration which has been done and from observing every one of these individuals stirring up bees with rosemary and mayonnaise and cushioning their heads with warm towels or setting on shower covers to hold the gunk of a wreck on, to find that whenever it has been flushed off and shampooed your hair is quite very much saturated and adapted, amazing!

Indeed, it was discovered that the fundamental fixing in these items is what your hair needs and that primary fixing are protein. This develops its fortitude, gives it more body and sparkle (with a couple of mystery fixings, all from your organizer, for example, nectar and olive oil). Another significant factor is the sort of food that we eat, as this guarantees that our hair is at its pinnacle condition.

1. A lot of protein in the eating regimen

2. A lot of water

3. Some state that coconut milk is also excellent for keeping up the sparkle, drinking, and utilizing it inside a combination of conditioner recipes.

These things can be found in our cabinets at home, so young ladies, on a Friday night, nothing to do, check around a couple of the recipes on the web and begin making your magnificent items which are unquestionably less expensive, and all the fixings will be natural where a portion of the items on the rack may somewhat contrast in their synthetic complexities and individuals would truly prefer not to put this on their hair. It is the all-natural young lady in age and the freshest items to guarantee the general natural look and feel.

The time is the factor in these customs made hair conditioners, and for the style cognizant, it would presumably be ideal to remain in because of the headgear or shower covers that should be worn.

Significant: Let individuals realize that you will require the shower room and make the night yours, watch a film! Be that as it may, it is the final product that is amazing. Through the retention and saturating of the hair follicles from the wonderful recipes, it is certainly perceptible. How awesome does anybody feel whenever they have been spoiled for the night?

NOTE: Do not be put off by the mayonnaise and how to apply it or what it resembles. Simply think about the outcome.

SUNFLOWER AND AMLA BEST NATURAL HERBAL HAIR CONDITIONERS

It is taken from Indian gooseberries, a local to South Africa. These natural items have different therapeutic and homegrown advantages connected to them, especially in hair care. Their utilization in treating hair related issues goes back to a huge number of years.

Amla oil has been utilized broadly as Ayurvedicmedicine to treat hair fall and turning gray and to shield hair from the harm that can occur because of residue and contamination. The oil has zero results and is the best natural homegrown hair conditioner that leaves your hair flexible, sparkling, and delicate.

As on account of Amla oil, Sunflower oil also is perceived for quite a long time as the best homegrown and restorative arrangement containing properties that fix different hair related issues, for example, hair misfortune and dandruff. The Sunflower oil likewise works viably as a hair conditioner. In this way, these two oils have been named the best natural homegrown hair conditioners.

Throughout the long term, the marvels of Sunflower and Amla have been known to mankind, and they have arisen as probably the best wellspring of homegrown cures in turning into natural homegrown hair conditioners.

Let us see a portion of the significant advantages of Amla and Sunflower oil that will demonstrate how plentiful they are.

1. Amla oil, whenever applied on the scalp, can forestall thinning up top and advance sound and peaceful rest. Amla oil is exceptionally valuable in upgrading memory and astuteness.

2. It can forestall, and now and again, even fix wrinkles to a degree.

3. This oil forestalls pressure, hence is additionally viable in forestalling maturing.

4. Amla oil gives a cooling impact on the head. That is one of the numerous explanations behind its broad utilization in nations, for example, India, where the atmosphere is hot and moist.

5. The Amla oil goes about as a natural hair conditioner restoring the scalp and keeping hair sound and sparkling for a more drawn-out length. It is additionally utilized for the avoidance of silver hair.

6. It advances the development of hair and forestalls pigmentation too.

7. Sunflower oil ensures hair misfortune by going about as a conditioner and emollient and nearly has all the properties of Amla oil.

One can undoubtedly dispose of hair issues rapidly with these compelling natural homes grown cures. Also, these natural cures are liberated from any results. Without much of a stretch, one can notice the distinction in the hair, utilizing these natural cures over a period.

Herbs and Spices

There is a motivation behind why herbs and spices have been utilized for quite a long time for pretty much anything, yet the restorative properties of herbs and so forth are by a wide margin their most noteworthy resource. Various herbs have various capacities and various qualities. There are wide assortments of herbs that animate the development of dark hair.

The greatest bit of leeway of utilizing herbs is that they are all-natural, and most are genuinely simple to discover. To sweeten the deal even further, herbs will, in general, smell truly pleasant regardless of what sort of oil is utilized as a base for medicines, veils, tonics, serums, and etcetera. The accompanying segments investigate the best herbs and spices to develop hair, forestall hair misfortune, and reinforce existing strands. Initial, a basic implantation formula:

OIL INFUSION OF ROSEMARY AND SAGE

Ingredient:

1 cup olive oil

1/4 cup rosemary leaves

1/4 cup sage leaves

Steps:

1) Create a twofold kettle by setting a metal or glass bowl over a quarter-full pot of bubbling water.

2) Mix the herbs and oil in the bowl over the warmth for 30 minutes.

3) Pour into a container sufficiently large to oblige the oil. Secure a square of cheesecloth over the mouth with an elastic band.

4) Tuck the container away in a warm, dull spot for around fourteen days. Mix the blend once every day. This timeframe will assist the herbs with implanting the oil

5) After about fourteen days, strain the oil into a spotless plastic or glass container for lasting stockpiling.

6) Use the oil as a treatment or for styling purposes. Store the oil in a dim spot to keep it new as far as might be feasible.

ALOE

Aloe is multi-skilled. It mollifies, relieves, cleans, and energizes hair development. What's more, it smells pleasant and is anything but difficult to track down, particularly in the late spring months when burn from the sun is predominant.

ALOE LEAVE-IN CONDITIONER

Ingredient:

1/2 cup water

1/2 cup Aloe Vera gel

10 drops tea tree oil

Steps:

1) Mix fixings in a shower bottle.

2) Spray in hair and brush to disseminate. Incredible for detangling twists! Catnip

In all honesty, catnip is an extremely famous spice utilized by people of color for quite a long time to develop hair, and they are legitimized in their commitment to this fixing.

Catnip helps keep hair solid and invigorates the hair to develop. To address your inquiry, catnip is a fluffy leaf from the mint family.

CATNIP HERBAL RINSE

Ingredient:

2 cups bubbling water

1 Tablespoon catnip

Steps:

1) Place catnip in a glass astound and pour bubbling water into it. Permit it the precarious for 20 minutes.

2) Strain the spice and let the fluid cool until it has arrived at your ideal temperature.

3) After shampooing and molding your hair, flush with the catnip fluid. Try not to flush out the wash.

CAYENNE PEPPER OIL

Ingredients:

1 cup olive oil

2 Tablespoons cayenne pepper

Steps:

1) Mix the oil and cayenne in a container.

2) Store the oil combination in a dim spot for ten days before utilizing it.

CAYENNE PEPPER AND CASTOR OIL TREATMENT

Ingredients:

A 16-ounce container of castor oil

1/2 huge jug of cayenne pepper

45 dark tea sacks

30 Biotin pills in powder structure

2-4 drops onion seed oil

1-2 drops garlic seed oil

Steps:

1)Preheat the stove to 200°F.

2)In a 2-quart heating dish, void the container of castor oil and the cayenne pepper.

3)Break open the tea sacks and empty the free tea into the dish.

4)Pop open the Biotin pills and add the powder to the blend.

5)Stir the blend completely, making a point to scratch sides. The blend will resemble a dark slime.

6)Bake in preheated broiler for 5 minutes, 30 seconds. Eliminate from broiler and coolenough to deal with.

7)Use nylon or cheesecloth to strain the combination into a jug.

8)Add the onion seed and garlic seed oils and shake to fuse.

CHAMOMILE HERBAL RINSE

Ingredients:

2 cups bubbling water

1 Tablespoon chamomile

Steps:

1)Place chamomile in a glass bowl and pour in the bubbling water. Permit it the lofty for 20 minutes.

2)Strain the spice and let the fluid cool until it has arrived at your ideal temperature.

3)After shampooing and molding your hair, wash with the chamomile. Try not to wash out the flush.

Natural Recipe Gel

NATURAL RECIPE GEL FOR HAIR WITH GELATIN

Gelatin contains keratin proteins, which combine with the hair to make them stronger. It holds fast, especially, to damaged areas and helps to smooth the nails' cuticle on the hair, helps to shine and reduce breakage.

However, you can get an overdose of something that is otherwise good. When I ate in this post about jelly hair, veils, firm hair are firm and adaptable, and hair with a lot of protein can stiffen, lose adaptability and become powerless against breakage. The extent of the jelly in this recipe is a bit to the point that it probably won't be a problem, regardless of whether you use it now and then; however, in case you see your hair losing its adaptability, it's a smart idea to take a deep state and turn this recipe into flaxseed or aloe

Ingredient:

1/4-1/2 teaspoon of gelatin (where to buy gelatin)

1/2 cup hot purified water

Up to 24 drops of essential oil (at your discretion)

Direction:

1. Divide the gelatin into warm water and use 1/4 teaspoon for a smaller take and 1/2 teaspoon for a larger take.

2. Include essential oils whenever you want. Store in a hermetically sealed stand in an icebox for up to 10 days.

ALOE VERA GEL FOR HAIR

Aloe vera is a great hair cream and scalp conditioner that also ends up as a styling gel. Several brands contain additives from which I want to maintain a strategic distance, but this is very acceptable.

Ingredient

1/2 cup aloe vera gel (this is the thing I use)

Up to 24 drops of essential oil (at your discretion)

Direction:

In using essential oils, add them to the aloe vera gel and mix to connect. Spot aloe in a hermetically sealed space. Since locally acquired aloe is established to extend the time frame of realistic applicability, this gel should be insisted at room temperature for three months.

RECIPE FOR FLAX HAIR GEL

Ingredient

3/4 cup refined water

1 tablespoon in addition to 1.5 teaspoons of flaxseed (where to buy flaxseed) up to 24 drops of essential oil

Direction:

1. Pour water and flaxseed into a saucepan and heat to a boiling point.

2. Reduce heat and simmer for about 10 minutes.

3. While the mixture is stewing, coat the grid filter with gauze.

4. When the liquid has stewed for 10 minutes, remove the pot from the oven and pour the liquid through gauze. At the moment when the liquid has separated, bring the edges of the gauze together and lift so that the flax seeds are at the bottom of the pocket (this should look like the pictures in the sketch of a newborn from the Stork transport) and barely get any remaining gel through the gauze with a couple of plates. (Try not to use your fingers because the liquid is extremely hot.)

5. Refrigerate for up to 10 days.

Healthy Hair With A Great Hair Rinse

Let us be honest. We, as a whole, need wonderful hair. It's absolutely not called "delegated magnificence" in vain - it does not just make you look great; it additionally causes you to feel great about yourself. Didn't somebody say that a lady finding the ideal hairdresser would say one is of life's most excellent things? This solitary shows the amount we esteem our delegated greatness - consequently, we need to deal with it and advance its wellbeing, much the same as we do with our bodies.

We are very much aware of the numerous items accessible for hair care. Shampoos, conditioners, and escalated medicines are on top of most records; however,we need excellent hair rinse to keep it sound.

For what reason Do We Need A Regular Hair Rinse?

Contamination, the sun's beams, solid shampoos, colors, dry air, and so on can make harm an extraordinary degree. This is the place where the significance of good rinse comes in. It takes the sparkle and life back to hair since it acts straightforwardly on our scalp instead of the hair shaft, where proteins and supplements are ingested.

Hair rinses reestablish the hair's natural PH balance. It attempts to explain hair - eliminating and last hints of shampoo or conditioner buildup. At the point when the explaining is done, our hair sparkles, and it gets milder! A decent rinse improves radiance and volume as well!

Furthermore, It likewise reestablishes the corrosive antacid equilibrium of our scalp. That corrosive soluble equilibrium is upset at whatever point we foolishly wash utilizing shampoos and get presented to chlorinated water.

The present formula utilizes herbs and lemons - how superb is that? Appreciate!

Vivacious LEMON and ROSEMARY HAIR RINSE

Ingredients:

1 new lemon

1 tsp. finely cleaved rosemary (for dim hair) or chamomile (for light hair)

1/2 cup of water

Directions:

1. Crush the lemon juice into a little bowl.

2. In a pan, put the finely hacked rosemary and pour in enough water to cover.

3. Heat to the point of boiling and stew for 5 minutes.

4. Strain the blend and let it cool.

5. Blend 2 tbsp. of the rosemary with the lemon juice in your bowl.

6. Pour this combination through your shampooed and molded hair.

7. Leave on the hair for 5 minutes.

8. Rinse hair completely with cool or lukewarm water.

Utilize this hair rinse once every week after shampooing and molding.

ROSMARINUS OFFICINALIS HAIR WASH RECIPE

Take two cups of refined water and include four tablespoons of rosemary. Heat the water till it decreases marginally. Strain the water and permit it to cool. In the wake of shampooing your hair, pour this wash over your hair. Utilizing fingertips gives the scalp a decent rub down also.

LEMON HAIR RINSE RECIPE

This hair Wash is ideal for individuals with light hair. To get a ready wash, join two cups of white vinegar, 2 cups of unadulterated refined water, one-quarter cup of newly crushed lemon juice, and a quarter cup of chamomile blossoms in a pan. Warm the fluid till it decreases slimly. Strain the fluid and keep it aside. Pour over the scalp and hair in the wake of shampooing. At last, Wash with cold water.

SAGE AND MALT HAIR RINSE RECIPE

In a polish bowl, mix two cups of malt, 2 cups of unadulterated refined water, and a quarter cup of sage. Warm the fluid till it decreases marginally. Move the bowl from the warmth source and strain the fluid. Take into consideration wash to chill off and afterward use it straightforwardly after shampooing the hair. At last, Wash the hair with cold water.

OCEAN KELP HAIR RINSE RECIPE

To set up this hair Wash recipe, make a lemon hair Wash, which will go about as the base. To the lemon hair Wash, include a quarter cup of ocean kelp, and blend in well. Next, exchange the wash to a container and handshake it energetically for 3 minutes. At that point, strain the fluid and pour it over shampooed hair. Wash it off with cold water.

TOMATO JUICE AND CORNSTARCH HAIR RINSE RECIPE

Consolidate one teaspoon of cornstarch with one cup of new tomato juice. Shampoo hair and pour wash. At last, Wash the hair with cold water.

NETTLE LEAF HERBAL HAIR RINSE

Nettle is the regular name for the plant Urticadioica, additionally called Stinging Nettle. Stinging Nettle herb is an excellent plant for reestablishing wellbeing and excellence to your hair. A herbal mixture produced using nettle leaf is a delicate and safe herb to rinse your hair with. It is additionally made into a mixture to drink each day. Indeed, you get greater sustenance to your entire body, skin and hair when you drink nettle implantation consistently and use it as a hair rinse week by week.

Nettle mixture takes a shot at within your body just as the outside. Plentiful in minerals and nutrients to support each framework in your body, nettles will cause your hair to develop, sparkle, get thick and obscure. A special reward is a smooth, clear skin and hard nails. Drink the implantation every day. Around 2-4 cups is the suggested sum. What's more, make additional implantation to use as a hair rinse.

Nettle mixture rinse eliminates parasitic and bacterial contaminations on the scalp. It helps balance an over-sleek skin or scalp, as well. Nettle stops hair misfortune and supports hair development. To make the hair rinse, simply make a quart of herbal implantation and use it as a rinse for your hair.

Instructions to make the implantation:

Put 1 ounce of dried nettle leaf in a quart glass canning container. Pour in bubbling water and mix to splash all the leaves. Cap with a cover and steep 2-4 hours. Drink day by day and use as a hair rinse once per week.

HEATING SODA RINSE

Try not to utilize this rinse any more than once per month to keep away from your hair's excessive drying. I know for a fact. It is truly powerful at eliminating any development of business items and can help balance your hair's pH levels.

To utilize this rinse, you will blend one tablespoon of preparing the soft drink in with one cup of warm water and rinse it through a few times. You do not have to clean this out. However, it is suggested if you have more obscure hair. In any case, the leftover preparing soft drink can make your hair look dull and fine.

CHAMOMILE TEA RINSE

Chamomile is a beautiful daisy-like herb that develops on fluffy green stems. This rinse will make light hair sparkle. There are two sorts of chamomile – Roman and German; it is possible that one can be utilized for this reason.

Start by making a tea; pour two cups of water over a quarter cup of new or dry chamomile blossom and let it steep until it is cool. Strain out the solids and use the fluid to rinse your hair multiple times. Leave the rinse in your hair.

HIBISCUS FLOWER RINSE

This rinse is useful for the fortunate rare sorts of people who sport red hair. On the off chance that you've ever picked a hibiscus blossom, you may have seen that it has some thick adhesive going through it. This is the thing that saturates your hair and draws out the ruddy features in it.

Use a quarter cup of new or dry hibiscus blossoms (new is ideal) and pour over two cups of bubbling water over the blossoms. Let it cool to room temperature before stressing out the solids. Rinse your hair multiple times; do not rinse this from your mind.

LEMON JUICE RINSE

You may figure your hair would be tacky when utilizing lemon juice, yet it is not. It has an incredible fragrance after washing. This rinse functions admirably for blondies and strawberry blondies since it can help your hair over the long haul. It will likewise free you of even the most difficult dandruff. It forestalls the breakage of the hair strand, as well.

You will require a quarter cup of new lemon juice, equal to the juice of a few lemons. Blend this in with 16 ounces of room temperature water. Shampoo your hair first, and afterward apply the rinse, rubbing it into your scalp and hair. Rinse at any rate multiple times; at that point, let your hair dry. Try not to get it in your eyes since it will consume.

The Best Recipe to style Hair

Giving an individual's hair repeatedly, look the cutting edge time of hairstyling utilizing different Hair Styling Tool. These assist in molding and extending the hair volume and subsequently causing the hair of an individual to show up shapely and energetic. Supermodels and different superstars advocate this in their hairstyles since this emphasizes their appearances and another body ascribes. This styling procedure of the renowned big names and design symbols has, throughout the years, streamed down to where a normal individual, with a bit, expertise, and capacity, can make similar styles in their own homes.

This can be refined by utilizing the advanced Hair Styling Tool that has hit the magnificence markets. These brushes have different shapes and sizes to oblige the different sorts of hair that exist in the human domain, from slim and long to thick and voluminous and can be bought by and large moderately modestly. The vast majority have styling look over for totally streamlining their hair or enumerating the hair in the wake of being styled with a coarse brush.

Among Professional Hair Styling Tool, the best varieties exist in the length and number of the individual "teeth" on the brush. These teeth are the determinant of how the hair is styled when utilizing the brush and can shift from being little and firmly stuffed in the plan of the brush to being enormous and separated. The size contrast in the teeth can make hair have a substantially more optimistic appearance or be extremely level and firmly stuffed to shield hair from looking rowdy.

The thicker teeth of styling brush permit the hair to be set up in an incredible number of higher plans that are mainstream among ladies today. Numerous ladies utilize hostile to static carbon brushes or pricey ionic imbued brushes that permit the hair to be liberated from static while searching to consider the hair's exact styling and plan. These styling brushes are exceptionally costly yet are accessible to general society in most magnificence flexibly shops or other excellent retail sources.

The coming of the crossbreed brush has been the most straightforward unrest of a styling brush. The brush's teeth are held in two distinct focuses and teeth styles, which makes it simpler to brush the hair into a more novel style with the assistance of one styling help. The hair can be completely smoothed, and the client will even now have the option to make a lifted style on different explicit zones on their head. A normal brush will not leave the hair alone styled from multiple points of view as a half and half brush.

A brush is a straightforward instrument that is yet utilized by numerous individuals to take a look that coordinates one's face and head. Even though there are numerous new hair styling items available, the brush is an apparatus that gives the client exactness and a customized look.

BEESWAX

Beeswax makes for a superb lip salve base. It's all-natural and, when applies, gives smooth and flexible lips. Numerous lip demulcents are comprised of oil and synthetic compounds that really dry out the lips instead of disguising dampness. A beeswax lip medicine will normally be bereft of hurtful synthetic substances and added substances.

Beeswax can likewise be utilized to make hair grease and mustache wax. On the off chance that looking for these items available, check the mark to guarantee that they are comprised of beeswax. Besides, beeswax can be utilized as a cream, like oil jam.

CHAMOMILE STYLING GEL

Additional hold. Fixes and makes diverse hairdo styles. Chamomile styling gel keeps your hairdo in its place the entire day with a natural appearance since it was uncommonly figured to make and fix distinctive hairdo styles. It is also the ideal supplement for the remainder of the chamomile styling gel Line, which naturally protects the blondness of the hair.

Wash your hair with shampoo and conditioner. Take the necessary measure of gel and apply it with the fingers on your wet or dry hair. For a wet hair appearance, style your hair, dries naturally. For dry hair appearance, style your hair with a hairdryer getting the alluring look.

CURL CREAM

Sheabutter and coconut oil are normal to presume with regard to DIY twist creams. This specific recipe utilizes both while joining aloe vera gel for the surface and invigorating essential oils for that additional oomph.

Ingredients:

Shea butter

Coconut oil

Apricot piece oil

aloevera gel

Rosemary essential oil

Chamomile essential oil

Directions:

Soften and combine the shea spread and coconut oil; at that point, let the liquefied blend cool in the fridge until it halfway sets.

Whip with a hand blender, add the apricot portion oil, at that point,keep blending.

Add the unadulterated aloe vera oil until it is totally blended (and add essential oils for a restoring aroma, as wanted).

Move to a bricklayer container and store it in a dry, clean spot.

FLAX HAIR GEL

Flax seeds strengthen hair and make them less prone to breakage due to unsaturated omega-3 fats.

You can prepare this hair gel by soaking a quarter cup of flaxseed in two cups of water and a tablespoon of aloe vera gel for six hours in any case. Drain all the mixture in a saucepan over high heat and heat to a boil. Reduce heat and let it brew for 10-15 minutes, stirring occasionally. Seeds begin to thicken. Be careful with the mixture and do not allow it to thicken excessively. Put a little on the spoon and tip marginally. On the chance that it rushes to the edge and quickly sinks, you need more time to stew. If you gradually dribble, it's over. In case it does not move, it is too thick, and you will have to add a little boiling water.

Each time, reaching the right consistency, turn the heat and strain into a glass container, removing the solids.

Allow the mixture to cool to room temperature before mixing in three or five drops of essential oil at your discretion. Drain this mixture in a hermetically sealed compartment. This saves seven days. On the off chance that you do not use

both in seven days, you can drain the gel into a 3D shaped plate of ice and freeze. When the 3D shapes are frozen, you can take them out in a cooler bag, take them out and unfreeze the block when you need it.

To use, focus on a modest amount of hands and apply to soaked or dry hair before styling.

HAIR CREAM

Nature gives us the most helpful and the best items to make us look more youthful, excellent and charming. This implies that every lady or young lady can utilize natural solutions to deal with her hair without much of a stretch and to protect its sparkle and thickness. Thus, in this article, you will figure out how to make hair cream at home utilizing modest natural ingredients.

Ingredients

2 Tablespoons shea spread (discover natural crude shea margarine here)

½ Tablespoon coconut oil (discover natural crude coconut oil here)

½ Tablespoon olive oil (locate a decent olive oil here)

¾ teaspoon jojoba oil (discover natural jojoba oil here)

¾ teaspoon sweet almond oil (discover natural sweet almond oil here)

½ Tablespoon unadulterated aloe vera gel (discover natural, unadulterated aloe gel here)

⅛ teaspoon Vitamin E oil (find non-GMO Vitamin E oil here)

15-20 drops of essential oils - I utilized 6 drops rosemary, 5 drops chamomile, 5 drops bergamot (locate the natural essential oils we utilize and suggest here)

Directions

Consolidate shea spread and coconut oil in a glass estimating cup or half-16 ounces bricklayer container. Dissolve in the microwave for a couple of moments, or utilize a stopgap twofold heater (fill a little pot with around 1-2 creeps of water and set glass holder inside, warming on low until softened).

Add remaining ingredients and mix well to blend. Move to a little, shallow tin with a top (this way).

Refrigerate for a few hours or overnight until the blend is cooled and set up. Eliminate from the fridge and permit it to come to room temperature beforeusing.

Store at room temperature (for a pleasant, smooth consistency) and use inside a month. Refrigerate any sum you can't use inside that time.

To Use

A tad of this styling cream goes far, so start with an extremely modest quantity when first utilizing it. Dunk clean fingers into the cream, rub a limited quantity into your hands and apply to hair that is just somewhat clammy or totally dry. (I have not had great outcomes when utilizing it on wet or moist hair.)

Flaxseed fortifies hair and renders it less inclined to breakage because of its Omega-3 unsaturated fats.

You can make this hair gel by splashing a quarter cup of flax seeds in two cups of water and one tablespoon of aloe vera gel for at any rate six hours. Empty the entire combination into a pot on high warmth and heat it to the point of boiling. Turn the warmth down and let it stew for 10 to 15 minutes, blending occasionally. The seeds will begin to thicken. Watch out for the blend, and do not let it thicken excessively. Put some on a spoon and tip it marginally. If it rushes to the edge and drops rapidly, it needs more stew time. On the off chance that it trickles off gradually, it is finished. If it does not move, it is excessively thick, and you will need to add a little boiling water.

Whenever you have arrived at the correct consistency, transform off the warmth and strain it into a glass bowl, disposing of the solids. Let the combination cool to room temperature before blending in three to five drops of essential oil of your decision. Empty this blend into a hermetically sealed holder. This will save for seven days. If you do not utilize that much in seven days, you can empty the gel into an ice 3D shape plate and freeze it. When the shapes are frozen, you can pop them out into a cooler sack, eliminating and defrosting a block as you need it.

To use, take a limited quantity on your hands and apply it to clammy or dry hair before styling.

Ultimate Guide To Avoiding Hair Loss

Hair misfortune (androgenetic alopecia) mentions an explanation of hair misfortune that is influenced by the androgen hormone, a hereditary tendency for thinning and maturation. Due to the fact that these hormones cause unhappiness of the hair, the treatment is susceptible quickly and significantly prevents the lack of hair.

Androgenic Hormones

All in all, typical men, including women, produce male hormones. Testosterone, DHT and dihydrotestosterone (DHT) are the best-known ones they produce. The male adrenal glands and balls produce androgens, and in women by their adrenal glands and ovaries. In both sexes, these hormones are significant, but they occur in different focuses and totals.

By the time the hair follicles are presented with DHT, the long-term hereditarily inclined individual develops androgenetic alopecia or the absence of female and male exemplary hair.

In particular, in the cells of the hair follicle, as in the bodies sebaceous, there are chemicals behind 5-alpha-reductase that are in high levels, changing in the course of testosterone, which is then transported to these areas with the blood and into DHT.

Fancy bad luck hair:

1. the individual's hair loss is obtained from the maternal side.

False. Hereditary features are one of the factors of the unhappiness of hair, they tend to be obtained from both the father and mother.

2. Regular haircut of hair will make it thicker.

False. Despite the fact that when the hair is cut, it looks stronger from the beginning, the next three days, or somewhere around, the hair would fall out, and new hair would develop, have similar measures as precut hair.

3. Wearing a hat can cause hair loss.

False. The hood can help by closing the sun's Rays. Even when wearing a cap for an extremely extended time, it can cause sebum to pick up due to temperature changes and react with cholesterol to make the sebum stiffen the thorn, which cut the oxygen course so that the hair will fall out.

4. DHT is the explanation of hair misfortune.

False. Even thoughthe overproduction of DHT is a huge purpose of unhappiness for the hair, it is not the main source.

5. Constant shampoo and hair drying lead to the unhappiness of the hair.

False. Heat can damage the hair; the purpose behind the weak hairdoes not hurt the basic foundation of the hair.

Shockingly more horrendous, some prescription drugs are known to cause hair hardship. Avoid expecting there is any opportunity of this occurrence the going with drugs:

Cholesterol-cutting down prescriptions:

- clofibrate (Atromis-S)

- gemfibrozil (Lopid)

- Antidepressants:

- tricyclics, amphetamines

High circulatory strain:

- atenolol (Tenormin)

- metoprolol (Lopressor)

- nadolol (Corgard)

- propranolol (Inderal)

- timolol (Blocadren)

Antithyroid:

- carbimazole

- Iodine

- thiocyanate

- thiouracil

Ulcer drugs:

- cimetidine (Tagamet)

- ranitidine (Zantac)

- famotidine (Pepcid)

- Anticoagulants:

- Coumarin

- Heparin

Moves you can make to thwart hair hardship:

- Stop concealing or perming your hair much of the time, for it can hurt it

- Limit introduction of your hair to chlorine

- Avoid distorted brushing or brushing wet hair

- Use a conditioner each after shampoo to make getting ready sensible and more straightforward

- Regulate heat introduction. Blow-drying, hot-turning and introduction to fixing irons may hurt your hair as time goes on

- Avoid drugs that can lead to hair incident, for instance, Vitamin A, testosterone things, beta-blockers, certain antidepressants and certain cholesterol-cutting down trained professionals

- Too much alcohol should be avoided. Be careful in picking your hair care things as some contain alcohol and add to hair dryness, delicate hair slanted to breakage.

- Tight ponytails and plaits can incite hair hurt

- Maintain a sound eating routine, eating heaps of verdant nourishments and drinking enough water

- Birth control pills can add to hair disaster

- Consult your PCP if should you notice peculiar hair mishap, as specific infirmities, for instance, lupus or having polycystic ovaries, or hyperthyroidism can cause hair incident

Supplements you can accept to hinder hair mishap:

- Thiamin (B1)

Containing the mineral sulfur, this is the essential segment of the hair that gives glimmer and shimmer.

- Riboflavin (B2)

This supplement is essential for body cell breathing, ensuring capable oxygen use for cell fix and creation.

- Niacin (B3)

Helps with enlarging vessels and vessels, thusly growing the bloodstream to the scalp to help energize hair advancement. It moreover may decrease the cholesterol create, which is essential since cholesterol on the scalp will change over to the compound 5 alpha-reductase.

- Pantothenic Acid (B5)

This supplement helpers in restoring hair tone and magnificence. It works with the amino destructive Tyrosine Folic Acid, PABA and Copper in the debilitation of white and silver hair.

- Biotin (B7)

Biotin is a comprehensively used fixing in hair things on account of its hair propelling properties. Biotin assembles hair cortex adaptability, thwarts breakage, and thickens hair fingernail skin.

- Cobalamin (B12)

Recuperates red platelets for sound hair.

- Pyridoxine (B6).

Liable for protein utilization balance, it helps in the delivery of amino acids to the right tissues. Moreover, this is essential in the difference in one amino destructive to another, like the change of Methionine to Cysteine. With Inositol, they control the oil stream to the scalp and the skin.

Conclusion

It may seem less difficult and more useful to buy excellent ready-made items to accelerate hair development. However, they may not be as strong as the items you can use at home. Each of these jars that cover the shelves contains synthetic substances, additives, and dozens of different components that you should not apply to your body.

Making your own hair development recipes at home can be a lot of fun; put aside the money, the ingredients are mostly natural and determine which recipe works for you. The "fun" perspective may not be so clear to some, in any case, see preparing a hair treatment such as conducting a scientific test or preparing dinner. Just put things in your head and get messy in the end!

At the finish, you could serve a considerable amount of money for a branded item or have an expensive salon treatment. The option is to follow a small amount of the cost of assembling the ingredients that you need to create yourself, and you will do it when it is convenient for you.

One of the best factors to make your hair development remedies is that the ingredients are quite natural. You can formulate every part of the recipe, and there is no need to think if you are doing more harm than anything to your hair. Doing this without someone else's help also gives you the opportunity to choose, Discard and change any recipe you use. You can have a go at everything you could want, and on the off chance that it does not work, you are only a few dollars away.

The fragrance is another motivation for a completely natural recipe made to measure. Some store brands smell good, but nothing better than the smell of a homemade fermented mixture, especially one that allows you to choose a fragrance that requires more. Finding a tonic, elixir or serum that works for you and makes your hair grow is the goal. This does not mean that you must give up the great ingredients for the brand planner.

Getting your hair to develop longer and fuller will not happen without any guile. No wonder the recipe mystically lengthen the hair in a few days. The way to grow hair is to discover a mixture that works for you. Some recipes' routine will probably be the ideal approach; however, the violation code and sort which recipes might be an instance of experimentation.

As you venture through your experimentation cycle, finding new ingredients and exploring different options when it comes to recipes, you will eventually find the right ones for you and work for your hair type and explicit hair they need. Regardless of anything else, all you need is some perseverance, stability, and market.

Printed in Great Britain
by Amazon